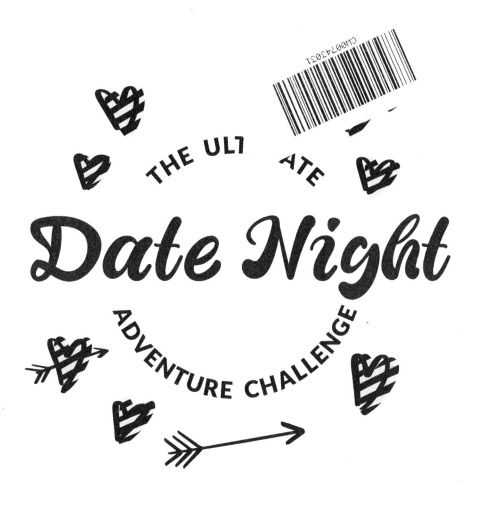

THE ULTIMATE
Date Night
ADVENTURE CHALLENGE

Over 100 Fun & Exciting Date Night Ideas
To Remember With Scrapbook Inside

Nicole Jones

Contents

PART II
NIGHTS OUT

PART III
TAKE ON THE CHALLENGE!

Introduction

How many times have you been on a date, only for it to turn out to be a complete disappointment?

Your date themselves might be perfectly fine, of course! The conversation might be flowing, the jokes and quips bouncing back and forth, and the plans for a second date being made. But the date itself—the choice of activity, the thing you decide to do, the restaurant or bar you drop in on—well, just falls flat.

Then again, maybe you're in a perfectly happy long-term relationship, but your date nights nowadays always tend to be the same kind of thing. Does that sound familiar?

You know the sort of thing. You go out for food here. You go out for a couple of drinks there. And every once in a while, you might go and catch a film, go for a walk in the country, or have a bit more of a lavish night out in a local bar or club. But when that turns out to be all you're doing on your date nights, week after week after week, even the best nights out and the best nights in can soon prove a little monotonous and more than a little boring!

So how about something a little bit more exciting, eh? Or, for that matter, how about 101 more exciting things? Happily, that's exactly where this book comes in!

This is *The Ultimate Date Night Adventure Challenge*—a collection of more than one hundred unique ideas specially compiled to make your next one hundred date nights a lot more fun, a lot more interesting, and a lot more exciting.

From fun games and activities to trying out new hobbies—and from ideas for nights in to ideas for days out—the next 100 pages are chock full of fascinating date night suggestions, many of which you might never have even thought of or considered otherwise. But there's something else that makes this book different.

As well as giving you dozens of new date night ideas, each page in this book has been specially arranged to allow you to scrapbook your dates as you try them out. So whether that means noting down your experiences or feelings afterwards, pasting in receipts or mementos from the activity in question, or even sketching your memories or printing out snapshots to keep in this book forever, page by page *The Ultimate Date Night Adventure Challenge* builds into a unique romantic scrapbook—letting you keep track of everything you and your date do, from start to finish!

There's also room on the pages here to rate these ideas and your date night experiences, on a scale of one to five hearts—one being a dud that doesn't quite fulfill expectations, and five being the perfect experience you'll be sure to try again! Use the "HOW DID IT GO?" part of the page to record how things went on the date and why you've awarded the date the score that you have.

That being said, of course, you should feel free to use all the open space on these pages to record whatever you want from your dates, no matter what memories or mementos they might be.

After all, these are your dates at the end of the day—and this is your Ultimate Date Night book!

PART I

Staying In

At-Home Movie Marathon

DATE: ____ / ____ / ____

Do you and your date have similar tastes in movies? Whether you do or you don't, click through to your favorite streaming platform or fire up the DVD player and pick out a night of cinematic entertainment together. It's up to you how you organize it—whether that means it's a romcom or tearjerker kind of night, or a hiding-behind-the-cushions horror marathon! Or perhaps pick out two movies each—so you can each impose your favorites onto the other whether they like it or not!

HOW DID IT GO?

_____

_____

_____

_____

_____

DATE RATING: ♡ ♡ ♡ ♡ ♡

Pasta Night

DATE: _____ / _____ / _____

Have you ever tried making your own pasta from scratch? It's a surprisingly (or perhaps deceptively) straightforward process! All you need to do is mix up a combo of flour, eggs, water, and oil by hand on a countertop, to make a dough dense enough that it can then be rolled, cut, twisted, or folded into whatever shape you like! A pasta night like this makes an excellent night in for foodies—giving you a chance to try or improve a new skill while preparing a (hopefully) delicious meal for yourselves... Just track down a simple beginners' recipe online, on YouTube, or in your favorite cookbook, and start getting your hands dirty!

HOW DID IT GO?

_____

_____

_____

_____

_____

DATE RATING: ♡ ♡ ♡ ♡ ♡

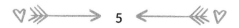

Portrait Painting

DATE: ____ / ____ / ____

No matter how artistic or creative you are, here's a fun idea for an arty night in. First, head to the local arts and crafts store to pick up some supplies— paints, brushes, pencils, charcoal, erasers, that kind of thing! Make sure too to pick up a couple of drawing pads or artist's canvases. Then, for your arty date night in, you and your date take a seat opposite one another and (perhaps with a glass of wine and some snacks alongside you!) draw one another. Make sure not to show your date your efforts until you're both done, of course—the big reveal at the end of the evening is all part of the fun...

HOW DID IT GO?

_____

_____

_____

_____

_____

DATE RATING: ♡ ♡ ♡ ♡ ♡

Draw a Relationship Comic Book

DATE: ____ / ____ / ____

Are you a talented artist? Are you and your partner budding Picassos? Not to worry if not, of course. This date night challenge idea works just as well (and often proves all the funnier!) if neither of you are particularly good drawers. The challenge is simply to draw, frame by frame, a comic book-style take on your relationship together or a moment from your past. No matter how long you've been a couple—or whether this is just one of your first few dates—drawing out, sketch by sketch, a series of comic recollections of, say, your first night out, your first Christmas together, or the time you met one another's parents or family is a fun way of both taking a trip down memory lane and giving each other a good laugh in the process.

HOW DID IT GO?

_____

_____

_____

_____

_____

DATE RATING: ♡ ♡ ♡ ♡ ♡

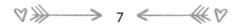

Try Bread-Making

No doubt partly inspired by the success of programs like *The Great British Baking Show*, a few years ago it seemed everyone everywhere was suddenly making their own farmhouse loaves and sharing pictures of their new sourdough starters! Whether you got swept up in that bread-making trend or not, attempting to make loaves of bread together is a fun date night idea no matter your experience! Simply track down a recipe online—or follow some tutorial steps on YouTube or some similar website—and either bake a single loaf together or tackle one each and have a taste test to see whose is the best. Be mindful of time, though—you don't want a recipe that's going to take you all day, so be sure to find something that you can get through in an evening (over a glass or two of wine, perhaps!).

HOW DID IT GO?

DATE RATING: ♡ ♡ ♡ ♡ ♡

Write Each Other a Poem

"Shall I compare thee to a summer's day?" William Shakespeare famously wrote, in one of the most romantic poems of all time. You might not square up to The Bard when it comes to tackling the ins and outs of poetry, but writing one another a short love poem is a fun date night activity nonetheless! It's up to you how seriously or how comically you tackle this one—and likewise, it's up to you to decide what aspect of your partner or your relationship you'd like to immortalize in verse. Will it be something as romantic as your first date or your first trip away together? Or would you rather tackle one of their annoying habits or bugbears? Whether it's a love sonnet overflowing with romance or a series of naughty limericks, grab yourselves a pad, a pen, and a writing dictionary, and get to work!

HOW DID IT GO?

_____

_____

_____

_____

_____

DATE RATING: ♡ ♡ ♡ ♡ ♡

Bake a Cake

If there's one thing the recent success of baking shows on television have shown it's how deceptively difficult successfully baking a cake can be! Everything has to be precisely measured, mixed, and combined, before being baked at just the right temperature for just the right amount of time. As tricky as it can undoubtedly be, though, baking a cake is a lot of fun—especially when you take it on together (or, for a nice competitive spin on this baking idea, bake a cake each to see whose comes out the best!) So why not track down a recipe online, stock up on all the necessary ingredients and equipment, and head to the kitchen to put your baking, frosting, and decorating skills to the test?

HOW DID IT GO?

DATE RATING: ♡ ♡ ♡ ♡ ♡

Terrible Movie Night

DATE: _____ / _____ / _____

When was the last time you went to the cinema and saw an absolute disaster of a movie? Or do you have a childhood favorite film that perhaps hasn't quite stood the test of time as you might like it to? Then again, is there a film that you absolutely love that your partner absolutely detests and loathes you putting on when you have a night in together?! Well, welcome to your Bad Movie Night! Get the popcorn and snacks, and pick one film each—the only rule being it has to be a so-bad-it's-good stinker of a movie. It might sound like a crazy idea, but watching a terrible film can make for a laugh-a-minute night in, so long as you and your other half go with the flow and make fun of how heinous the whole thing is. No idea what to watch? Why not track down a list of Hollywood's worst movies online and go from there…

HOW DID IT GO?

_____

_____

_____

_____

_____

DATE RATING: ♡ ♡ ♡ ♡ ♡

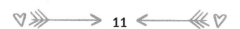

Cook a Three-Course Meal

DATE: _____ / _____ / _____

We're heading back into the kitchen for this one, only this time we're taking on that most important restaurant staple: the three-course meal! First, you and your partner need to decide on a menu—that is, starter, main course, and dessert. Then you need to decide how you're going to split up the cooking. Are you both going to work on every course, or would you rather one handles the starter, the other the entrée, and you dish out the dessert together? You can be as adventurous and as formal as you like here, too. Why not chill the wine and get some appetizers on the go for a sophisticated fine-dining experience—or, if that's not quite your style, why not go for the ready-made options, keep the cooking to a minimum, and chill out on the sofa while the microwave does all the hard work? Whether it's a black tie or pajamas kind of evening, put your culinary skills to the test together!

HOW DID IT GO?

_____

_____

_____

_____

_____

DATE RATING: ♡ ♡ ♡ ♡ ♡

Write a "Consequences" Story

DATE: ____ / ____ / ____

Have you ever played a game of Consequences? If you haven't, it works a little like this: set a timer running for, say, anything from 30 seconds to a minute. Then, you and your partner grab a pen and a piece of paper each and begin writing a story. (This being a date night challenge, of course, it's only fitting that you two should be the main characters in one another's tales, so be sure to include lots of personal details and inside jokes!) Once the timer runs out, stop writing—regardless of whether it's midsentence or still only a few lines in!—and fold the paper back so that only the last few words or lines can be seen. Then pass your paper to your partner and vice versa, and start the timer again, with both of you picking up the other's story from where they left off. After a few passes back and forth, bring your stories to a close, unfold your papers, and then see where your imaginations have taken you!

HOW DID IT GO?

_____

_____

_____

_____

_____

DATE RATING: ♡ ♡ ♡ ♡ ♡

Plant a Tree Together

This one's a fun one for the spring and summer months. Head down to your local garden center or outdoors store, and pick up a young potted tree or sapling. Then head home (if you're lucky enough to have a yard or some outside space at your house!) and take the time together to give the newest addition to your garden it's new start in life. As well as being a lot of fun and some good outdoor exercise, this can be a surprisingly touching activity—especially if you coincide planting your tree together with your anniversary, or one another's birthdays. Not to worry if outdoor space isn't available at home, though. You can always move this activity indoors and have an evening of potting plants or flowers, or even put together a mini herb garden for your kitchen window sill—why not?

HOW DID IT GO?

_____

_____

_____

_____

_____

DATE RATING: ♡ ♡ ♡ ♡ ♡

Write a Couple's Quiz

Who doesn't like a good quiz game or a trivia night? Well, for the odd date night in, writing your own couple's quiz can be a fun way both of reminiscing about your time together and picking up on each other's quirks and eccentricities! The idea behind it is simple. Each of you writes a series of questions (say, 10 or 20, or so), and then you quiz one another to see if your partner can work out the answer. You can make this as tricky, as personal, and as comical as you like. So if you're the kind of person who tends to remember the finer details of your past nights out—such as precise dates, restaurant names, what you were wearing, and so on—perhaps this might be a good opportunity to test your partner's memory of those? Especially if they're *not* the kind of person who tends to remember that kind of thing…!

HOW DID IT GO?

_____

_____

_____

_____

_____

DATE RATING: ♡ ♡ ♡ ♡ ♡

Track Your Family History

Family history research has seen something of a boom in interest in recent years, thanks to the success of documentary programs like *Who Do You Think You Are?* and *Finding Your Roots*. It can take months, if not years, to track down and map out a full family tree, of course, so that's a little beyond what you might be able to figure out in just an average date night in! But drawing up your and your partner's family trees as far as you can is a great way of finding out more about one another. Be sure to open this up to family members too, of course—why not drop a few messages to parents or aunts and uncles and see how far back and how far outwards you can draw those family ties?

HOW DID IT GO?

DATE RATING: ♡ ♡ ♡ ♡ ♡

Play a Taste Test Game

DATE: ____ / ____ / ____

This is a fun at-home game idea that you can make as crazy or as delicious as you like! All you have to do is arrange some kind of taste test for your partner. Perhaps it might be something ordinary, such as pasta sauces, soups, sodas, or dips. Or perhaps you might like to go a little more off the wall and throw two random ingredients into the mix and see if your partner can tell the two mismatched foodstuffs you have Frankensteined together! This game works even better if you're blindfolded and you can't pick up on any clues like the color or appearance of what you're tasting! So whether you're being nice—and naming something like fresh fruits, salad dressings, or smoothies—or gruesomely raiding the kitchen cupboards for some awful mix of barbecue sauce and breakfast cereal, get a blindfold at the ready and get serving!

HOW DID IT GO?

_____
_____
_____
_____
_____

DATE RATING: ♡ ♡ ♡ ♡ ♡

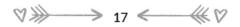

How Much Do You Really Know?

So we've already tried out a trivia night here, but how about this for a spin on a traditional question and answer quiz: instead of asking questions about how much you can remember about your time together or about one another's quirks and eccentricities, each of you should write a quiz about yourself. Then, question by question, ask your quiz and see how much your other half really knows about you. Quiz them on things like your first pet's name or your first car. Your favorite color, your favorite high school subject, or your favorite movie, album, or actor. Why not ask them to name some of your extended family members or extended circle of friends? Or how much do they really know, for instance, about what you keep in your glove compartment, the attic, or the cupboard under the stairs?!

HOW DID IT GO?

_____

_____

_____

_____

_____

DATE RATING: ♡ ♡ ♡ ♡ ♡

Try Origami

Origami is the beautiful and ancient Japanese art of making delicate geometric models out of squares of paper. It can take years to master, unsurprisingly, and true origami experts can make folded versions of everything from honeybees to water birds! Not to worry if that's not quite where you're starting from, of course, because learning origami together is a great way of testing one another's creativity on an otherwise quiet date night in. You're going to need paper for this one and it might be worth heading to a craft store for some proper origami paper, which is typically a little lighter than regular paper to make the folds easier and sharper. You might even be able to track down an origami kit there if you're lucky, but not to worry if you can't—you can easily cut regular A4 paper down to size and follow instructions and tutorials online!

HOW DID IT GO?

_____

_____

_____

_____

_____

DATE RATING: ♡ ♡ ♡ ♡ ♡

Learn to Juggle

Here's a real test of your coordination and motor function—learning to juggle! Don't worry, we're not quite going to leap ahead to burning clubs or torches just yet. Instead, get yourself a set of three or four matching balls, pompoms, or even squares of fabric (which are lighter, and so don't move quite so quickly through the air—making them easier to keep track of and catch!). Then, load up a juggling tutorial online and see which one of you is the first to manage keeping three—and then maybe even four or more!—balls or squares in the air at the same time. Juggling is a lot harder than it might appear, of course, so don't be too downhearted if you're not an expert right away! Though best to start practicing nowhere near any vases or priceless family heirlooms...

HOW DID IT GO?

DATE RATING: ♡ ♡ ♡ ♡ ♡

Break a World Record

DATE: ____ / ____ / ____

Every year, thousands of new world records are set and broken all over the world. Not all of them are quite as serious and as immediately impressive as a new 100m sprinting time, however, and we're not suggesting you tackle anything too wild on a quiet date night in! Instead, first of all, pick an activity that you think you're good at—or else, that you think you *might* be good at. Hula hooping. Pancake flipping. Envelope stuffing. Memorizing a shuffled deck of cards, that kind of thing. Then, have a quick search online (all the official Guinness World Records are listed on their website!) and find out what the current world record is. Can you match it, get anywhere near it—or even break it?! Set the timer running and find out...

HOW DID IT GO?

Make a Time Capsule

It's something that's better associated with high school history projects and new civic developments. But making a time capsule together can be a sweet, fun, and fascinating date night activity—both now, and in the future. It's up to you how you handle this, of course, and where exactly you wish to leave your time capsule for posterity. Perhaps you'd just like to write your future selves letters, and then—without looking—place them in an envelope to be kept somewhere safe until, say, some anniversary down the line when what you have written has all but slipped from your memory. Or perhaps you'd like to go the whole hog—putting photographs, souvenirs, and other items (nothing perishable, of course!) into a lockbox and keeping it out of sight until the agreed time to open it arrives.

HOW DID IT GO?

DATE RATING: ♡ ♡ ♡ ♡ ♡

"First Word" Challenge

DATE: ____ / ____ / ____

If I were to say to you the word BARBECUE, for instance, what is the first word that comes to mind? Or what if I were to say HOLIDAY or BREAKFAST? Or how about NIGHTMARE, PHOBIA, or TERRIFYING? Playing a game of First Words on a date night in can be a fun way of finding out how well you know each other—and how the other person's brain ticks! To play, all you have to do is to come up with a prompt word, just like those above, and then write down what you think will be the first word that your other half will think of when you say it to them. It's up to you what prompts you use, of course, and you can make a start with those above—but the more personalized your prompts are, the more fun (and more revealing!) this game can be!

HOW DID IT GO?

_____

_____

_____

_____

_____

DATE RATING: ♡ ♡ ♡ ♡ ♡

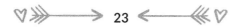

Have an At-Home Picnic

DATE: ____ / ____ / ____

You don't have to wait for a fine summer's day to have a picnic. Instead, a quiet night in can be the perfect opportunity to make yourselves a meal in a basket and chill out together. The idea is simple—pack whatever you would normally take to a picnic in the park or in the countryside into a satchel or a basket, then spread a blanket out on the living room floor and enjoy! Bizarrely, this idea works brilliantly in the depths of winter, or even around Christmas or New Year, when the weather outside might be the complete opposite of picnic weather! Instead, snuggle up with your snacks, fruit, sandwiches, and sweet treats in front of the fire, and have an indoor picnic at home!

HOW DID IT GO?

DATE RATING: ♡ ♡ ♡ ♡ ♡

Play a Board Game

DATE: ____ / ____ / ____

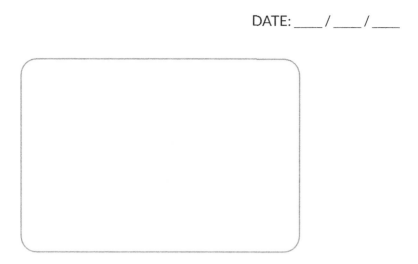

In this day and age of online games and apps, the simple pleasure of playing a classic dice-rolling, counter-moving, question-asking board game might not be high on many people's agenda when it comes to relaxing at home. But picking a fun board game to play at home and challenge one another to is a great hands-on alternative to endless scrolling and playing on your cell phone or tablet. Simply pick a game of your own choice—perhaps an endless classic like Trivial Pursuit or Scrabble, or else something you've never played or tried before—and with some snacks and drinks at your side, get playing!

HOW DID IT GO?

_____
_____
_____
_____
_____

DATE RATING: ♡ ♡ ♡ ♡ ♡

Try Indoor Gardening

DATE: ____ / ____ / ____

From potted plants to window boxes and kitchen herb gardens, the options for growing your own greenery at home—even without the luxury of a back yard or lawn—are brilliantly varied. So how about getting your green thumbs dirty and trying out a little indoor gardening on your next date night in? It's up to you how this idea pans out, of course. You might want to try growing something from seed and seeing whose plant sprouts first or produces the first fruits or flowers on the window sill. Then again perhaps you might like to buy some potted herbs from the supermarket and try cultivating your own herb garden of thyme, rosemary, or basil in your kitchen. Then again maybe you want to buy a host of different smaller plants, and try potting them together as an indoor display. Decide what direction you want to go in, get your supplies, and get potting!

HOW DID IT GO?

_____

_____

_____

_____

_____

DATE RATING: ♡ ♡ ♡ ♡ ♡

Hobby Swap

DATE: ____ / ____ / ____

From playing an instrument or a video game to something as calm and creative as knitting, quilting, cross-stitching, and needlecraft, everyone has the one thing that they like to do to wind down. But how about swapping your favorite hobby with your partner for the night, and see how they get on? This challenge often proves all the more fun for couples whose favorite hobbies and pastimes are vastly different—such as seeing how someone who likes wood turning in the garage takes to making a patchwork quilt (and vice versa!). But no matter how similar or how seemingly boring or understated your favorite thing to do in your down time might be, taking the time to share and try out one another's hobbies is always a great way of seeing how your partner ticks!

HOW DID IT GO?

_____

_____

_____

_____

_____

DATE RATING: ♡ ♡ ♡ ♡ ♡

Plan the Perfect Trip

DATE: _____ / _____ / _____

Imagine money was no option. Your lottery numbers have finally come up. Some obscure, well-to-do long-lost relative has left you everything in their will. And imagine too that there's no work to go to tomorrow. You have nothing in your calendar, a clear schedule for weeks—if not months—to come. So, where are you going to go? Spend the evening planning the greatest trip imaginable with your partner, and let your imaginations run wild. It doesn't matter how far-flung your ideal destination (or destinations!) might be. It doesn't matter how long it might take to get there, how long you're staying there, or how expensive the travel might be. This is your perfect dream trip—going wherever you want, for however long you like. Why not even take a look online and see what five-star hotels, restaurants, and resorts you might hit up when you get there? And who knows, maybe one day you will!

HOW DID IT GO?

_____

_____

_____

_____

_____

DATE RATING: ♡ ♡ ♡ ♡ ♡

Play a Game of Song Tag

DATE: ____ / ____ / ____

How often do you and your partner listen to the same music? Most couples might have one or two artists or groups in mind that they both enjoy listening to, but there's often just as many more songs and artists that you and you alone tend to listen to at home! Song Tag is a great game to share your musical taste with your partner, and see if you can win them over to some artists or groups they might always have ignored! The rules are simple: you each take turns selecting a single song that you love and that you think the other person will enjoy, and play it in full. Once that song is complete, you tag your partner, and they get to play you *their* song of choice. Back and forth you go, one after the other, song after song! And who knows, perhaps you'll have a few new favorites to listen to once the evening is over?

HOW DID IT GO?

_____

_____

_____

_____

_____

DATE RATING: ♡ ♡ ♡ ♡ ♡

Play "Would You Rather...?"

Would you rather only be able to eat your favorite food once again for the rest of your life, or have to eat one serving of your least favorite food every week? Would you rather be stuck in an elevator with someone you hate for one hour, or stuck in an elevator on your own all day? And would you rather have to relive your first day of high school, or your worst day at work? Would You Rather is a classic game, of course, but playing it with your partner can be a fun way of picking up on things you know they love and hate, and finding out how they tick. Be sure to put together options that you know will tap into their likes and dislikes, and make the choices put in front of them as tricky as possible!

HOW DID IT GO?

_____

_____

_____

_____

_____

DATE RATING: ♡ ♡ ♡ ♡ ♡

Host an At-Home Drive-In

DATE: ____ / ____ / ____

The drive-in movie theater isn't quite as common as it once was, of course, but there's little denying its place in American culture, and—thanks to Hollywood movies!—how quintessentially attached it is to the classic first date. If there's no drive-in nearby, or the weather isn't quite suitable for an outdoor cinema, however, not to worry—you can replicate the experience at home using a little bit of inexpensive gadgetry! These days, you can attach portable projectors to smart phones, tablets, and laptops, and with a white sheet hung on the wall you can replicate the cinema experience in the comfort of your own home. It's up to you to decide what this evening's showing is, of course—but there's no need to limit yourself to Hollywood movies! Why not try a showing of your vacation snapshots or clips from your favorite YouTuber or TikToker? Get the popcorn heating up, fire up the cinema, and park up on the sofa!

HOW DID IT GO?

_____

_____

_____

_____

_____

DATE RATING: ♡ ♡ ♡ ♡ ♡

Play a Card Game

Card games have been popular for as long as there have been decks of cards—and the very first of those were invented around one thousand years ago! As old-fashioned and as old-school as it might sound, why not try setting aside a night for a few rounds of your card game of choice? That being said, you don't have to limit yourselves to a game you both already know. Why not take a look online or in some compendium of games and pastimes and see how quickly you can pick up the rules of a new game from scratch? There's a wealth of fun card games, both old and new, just waiting to be discovered! So take a seat at the table, shuffle the deck, and get playing ...

HOW DID IT GO?

_____

_____

_____

_____

_____

DATE RATING: ♡ ♡ ♡ ♡ ♡

Play "Truth or Dare?"

DATE: ____ / ____ / ____

It's likely a game that you were more accustomed to playing in childhood at sleepovers or summer camps, but playing a few rounds of Truth or Dare? with your other half can be a hilarious way of finding out more about them. And, just like Would You Rather, be sure to make your truths (and your dares, for that matter!) as personalized as possible. So make sure to pick up on your partner's quirks and eccentricities, their likes and dislikes, and the people in their lives they love and love to hate! How daring you go, of course, is up to you—but remember, for every Truth or Dare you come up with, you're going to have to answer one in return!

HOW DID IT GO?

_____

_____

_____

_____

_____

DATE RATING: ♡ ♡ ♡ ♡ ♡

Have a Clear Out

It might not sound like the most fun activity in the romantic calendar, but a good household clear-out of all your long-unused junk and old clothes can actually make for a fun evening in! Pour a couple of drinks, decide what overstuffed area of the house you're going to tackle (the kitchen drawers and cupboards, or the dreaded back of the upstairs closet, for instance!) and see what you can set aside for a yard sale or to send to Goodwill. As you dig through all your old things, of course, you'll doubtless start to remember the tales and stories attached to them—and that's where this idea comes into its own. Whether it's the unwanted juice-pressing machine your partner's mother bought you for your birthday or your long-forgotten childhood schoolbag or soft toy, there can be a wealth of anecdotes and hilarity hidden away in your closets and cupboards!

HOW DID IT GO?

DATE RATING: ♡ ♡ ♡ ♡ ♡

Christmas Comes Early!

DATE: ____ / ____ / ____

Who doesn't love Christmas? It is, after all, The Most Wonderful Time of the Year! So why not make it come early, this year? No matter the date (and no matter the weather!), don your favorite festive sweaters, get some mulled wine on the stove, crank up the Mariah Carey, and have a fully festive night in! This works especially for couples that, due to work or family commitments, often end up having to spend Christmas apart. But whether you're able to have Christmas together or not, taking the time to celebrate the goodness in the world—and buying a little gift for one another as a token of your love and happiness together—has got to be worthwhile doing at any time of year!

HOW DID IT GO?

_____

_____

_____

_____

_____

DATE RATING: ♡ ♡ ♡ ♡ ♡

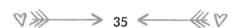

Learn Magic

Have you ever been to see a magician or an illusionist? It's quite incredible what truly talented performers and prestidigitators are able to do on stage— but they all have to start somewhere, and tonight is the night you're going to join them! Learning magic tricks is a hilarious opportunity to pick up a potential new skill while amazing one another with your new-found feats of illusionism. You can either track down tricks online (there are lots that you can easily do at home with an assortment of household objects, like a deck of cards, a few sheets of paper, or a book of matches), or else go all out and pick up a beginner's magic set from your local toy store and follow the instructions inside. The only rule is that you have to learn your tricks individually, and then perform them for one another. Can your partner figure out the secret? Or will you prove such a natural performer that they'll have no clue how you managed it?!

HOW DID IT GO?

_____

_____

_____

_____

_____

DATE RATING: ♡ ♡ ♡ ♡ ♡

Play Friends and Family Tag

DATE: ____ / ____ / ____

Do you have a favorite story about growing up with your family or one of your best friends? Have you ever told that story to your partner before? Friends and Family Tag is a great back-and-forth game for a date night in, in which you each take turns telling the funniest, daftest, or most heartwarming stories about the nearest and dearest people in your lives. Simply pick a tale from your past that you don't think you've ever shared with your partner before—perhaps it's something that happened with an old friend who no longer lives close by, or something an old family member got up to years ago when you were just a child—and tell it to them. Once your story is complete, it's their turn to tell you a tale, and back and forth you go from there, raiding the family histories for the quirkiest stories you can come up with!

HOW DID IT GO?

DATE RATING: ♡ ♡ ♡ ♡ ♡

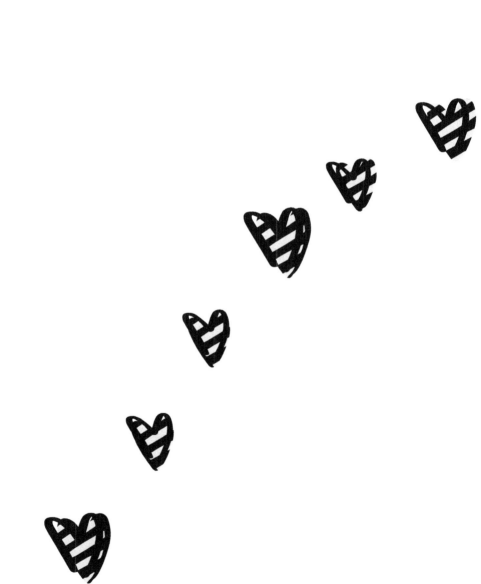

PART II

Nights Out

Casino Night

Chips down, cards at the ready! If you've never tried it before, why not head out for a night at the casino? Whether it's craps or roulette—and whether your bets are just a couple of dollars or something more eyewatering!—experiencing a casino is another life box ticked. Even if betting and wagering isn't for you, many casinos are as much up-market bars as they are gambling houses, so there is still much to enjoy and to experience even if you're just soaking up the atmosphere together! So there's just one more question left to answer—are you putting it on red or black?!

HOW DID IT GO?

_____

_____

_____

_____

_____

DATE RATING: ♡ ♡ ♡ ♡ ♡

Old Movie Night

DATE: ____ / ____ / ____

We've looked at a couple of options for at-home movie experiences already here, but there are few things more romantic that old Hollywood movies— and there are few places more romantic to experience them in than an old arthouse cinema. Take some time to track down a cinema in your area that specializes in showing the Hollywood greats, and get yourselves booked in for a night of Bogart and Bacall. Finding an old arthouse cinema might be easier said than done, of course, so this might be something that you need to factor into a trip further afield. But once you've got a venue in mind, finding the time to enjoy the best of Golden Age Hollywood can make for a romantic night that won't be forgotten.

HOW DID IT GO?

_____

_____

_____

_____

_____

DATE RATING: ♡ ♡ ♡ ♡ ♡

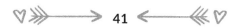

Re-enact Your First Date

Can you remember your first date together? Of course you can! So, whether it was only a matter of months or more a matter of years ago, how about recreating that very first meeting one evening together? Try to be as accurate as possible in your re-enactment. Can you remember how you had your hair, and what clothes you were wearing? If you went for food, can you remember the table you sat at or what part of the bar you happened to meet in? Or perhaps you met one another at a party, or a friend's house—in which case, why not open your re-enactment up to friends and family and bring everyone together for a night celebrating your time together?

HOW DID IT GO?

DATE RATING: ♡ ♡ ♡ ♡ ♡

Karaoke Night

DATE: ____ / ____ / ____

The karaoke craze might not be quite at the heights it was in the 1990s today, but a karaoke night is still a night on which fun and laughs are all but guaranteed! If you're able to book yourself a booth at a dedicated karaoke bar, of course, then organizing this one is going to be a piece of cake. If that's not an option, however, why not head down to your local bar or nightclub the next time they have a karaoke night on? Or failing that, why not track down a karaoke machine yourself to rent or buy, and host a fun night of singing along to your favorite tunes at home with your nearest and dearest? (Just maybe warn the neighbors first!)

HOW DID IT GO?

_____

_____

_____

_____

_____

DATE RATING: ♡ ♡ ♡ ♡ ♡

Amusement Arcades

It might not be something you've thought about doing since you were a child, but heading out to the amusement arcades at your local funfair or shopping mall is a sure-fire evening of fun and—quite literally!—games. As fun as retro classics like Frogger and Pac Man can be, of course, this doesn't just have to be video games. Traditional funfairs and carnivals will often have old school games to try out too, such as target darts and pellet-shooting ranges, water-cannon games (who can pop the clown's balloon the fastest?), and roll-a-ball games (in which you have to target your balls into slots on a sloped range, with moving wooden horses keeping track of everyone's score!). And while you're there, how about picking up some cotton candy and popcorn too?

HOW DID IT GO?

_____

_____

_____

_____

_____

DATE RATING: ♡ ♡ ♡ ♡ ♡

Escape Room

A few years ago, these were barely even a thing. Now escape room experiences can be found in practically every big city—and, so long as you're with the right people (and have a knack for solving puzzles!) are doubtless going to give you an intense hour or so of nerve-jangling fun. So why not track down a local venue and get yourself booked in? Who knows, you might turn out to be a natural clue-solver or code-cracker and figure your way out within a matter of minutes? Then again, perhaps that all depends on who you take into the room with you, and if it's just you and your partner—with no friends to bounce ideas off or to help you crack the games—perhaps it might be worth clearing your evening!

HOW DID IT GO?

DATE RATING: ♡ ♡ ♡ ♡ ♡

Take the Tourist Trail

DATE: ____ / ____ / ____

When you grow up or live in a place for a long time, it's often easy to take what it has to offer for granted. Every town and city of a decent size will have its own version of a tourist trail or walking tour, and no matter how long you've lived there, joining up with a tour group or going for a walk around your city's biggest and best sites can be a fun way of reminding one another of just how great a home you have on your doorstep! Whether you decide on cultural highlights, like galleries or museums, or something more outdoorsy—wandering the parks or heading up to a viewpoint, perhaps—seeing your home town together through a tourist's eyes can make for a day or a night to remember.

HOW DID IT GO?

_____

_____

_____

_____

_____

DATE RATING: ♡ ♡ ♡ ♡ ♡

New Outfit Challenge

DATE: ____ / ____ / ____

Shopping for new clothes down at the mall is often either someone's idea of perfect retail therapy, or their idea of the day from Hell! So how about this for a neat (and often unexpectedly hilarious!) twist on it? Together, you and your partner head to the local department store or shopping mall, and—with a strict budget in mind—pick out an entirely new outfit for the other person. Everything from socks and shoes upwards needs to go in the basket, before you head to the changing rooms to try it on. Perhaps there's a color or a style you've always wanted to see your partner wear that they've been hesitant to try? Or perhaps you just want to prank them and pick out an outfit, head to toe, you know they'll hate?! No pressure to buy anything at the end of the challenge, of course!

HOW DID IT GO?

_____
_____
_____
_____
_____

DATE RATING: ♡ ♡ ♡ ♡ ♡

Bowling Night

Whether you're a ten-pin master or not, heading out for a night at the local bowling alley is always a fun option. With food, snacks, and a few drinks on the go, get yourself booked in and see how well you do! And if there's something of a disparity between how natural a bowler you and your partner are, then why not make things interesting by playing to a handicap—doubling the weaker player's score along the way, perhaps, or adding any pins the other player leaves standing onto their score? Or how about inviting some friends or family members along and playing as two team captains? That way, you can spread the skillfulness equally between the two of you!

HOW DID IT GO?

_____

_____

_____

_____

_____

DATE RATING: ♡ ♡ ♡ ♡ ♡

Go-karting

DATE: ____ / ____ / ____

Another activity that might be all too closely associated with kids' parties and childhood memories, why not get yourselves booked in for a few laps at a local go-karting track? If you're unsure of how natural a karter you might be (or are worried that your partner will be far better than you!), remember that many tracks these days offer taster sessions and even trackside tuition with instructors and other drivers—so you can really make the most of the day, and not only challenge one another but practice an entirely new skill! By all means open this up to other couples and friends and family to make more of the day, of course—or else just keep it between the two of you and see who crosses the finish line first!

HOW DID IT GO?

_____
_____
_____
_____
_____

DATE RATING: ♡ ♡ ♡ ♡ ♡

Try a Wreck Room

Here's an activity that you've not only likely never tried, but might not even have heard of before! A craze since the early 2010s, wreck rooms are highly protected areas where you and your partner or friends can go and make as much mess and noise as you like without anyone being bothered! Wreck rooms will arm you with the likes of china plates and fake vases and glassware, as well as an array of hammers, wrenches, clubs, and sledgehammers—and all the necessary safety equipment too, of course!—before letting you loose in a totally safe and protected space. Smash up anything and everything you can find, knowing that no one is going to bat an eye (or give you a bill for the damage!). This is a great way of not only working up a sweat and having a great deal of fun but letting off some steam too.

HOW DID IT GO?

_____

_____

_____

_____

_____

DATE RATING: ♡ ♡ ♡ ♡ ♡

Go on a Nature Hike

DATE: _____ / _____ / _____

There's no denying that a little time outdoors in the fresh air is good for both your mental and physical health. So why not take some time to enjoy the natural world by heading out on a nature hike? Choose a local route that suits your experience and fitness levels (and choose a day on which the weather is on your side), then pack a bag and head out there. Be sure to follow all the usual rules here, of course: dress appropriately for whatever the weather may be, and make sure to pack something to eat and, in hot weather especially, plenty to drink. Rules followed, though, there's nothing more to do than enjoy nature in all its glory on a romantic day out in the wilderness!

HOW DID IT GO?

_____

_____

_____

_____

_____

DATE RATING: ♡ ♡ ♡ ♡ ♡

Picnic in the Park

Packing a basket of sandwiches, snacks, sweet treats, and a pitcher of ice-cold fruit juice (or perhaps something stronger!) and heading out to the park is a great way to casually spend a lazy spring or summer's afternoon together. Depending on the weather and the time of year, it might be difficult to find a quiet spot to yourselves, but once you're sorted, laying out a blanket on the cool grass—perhaps in the summertime shade of a tree alive with birds and bees—is surely one of life's simplest and most romantic pleasures!

HOW DID IT GO?

_____

_____

_____

_____

_____

DATE RATING: ♡ ♡ ♡ ♡ ♡

Theme Park

DATE: _____ / _____ / _____

Are you a rollercoaster kind of person, or more of a carousel kind of person? Are you going to be found queueing up for the water slide, or for the Ferris wheel? And is it going to be five minutes battling one another in the bumper cars, or a more leisurely paddle around the lake in a pedalo boat? No matter what your idea of the best day out at a theme park might be, taking the time to visit one together is a great way of letting off some steam, taking your mind of your troubles—and, of course, forcing one another to do the most adrenaline-pumping things you can find on offer! Simply track down your park of choice and make a day of it!

HOW DID IT GO?

_____
_____
_____
_____
_____

DATE RATING: ♡ ♡ ♡ ♡ ♡

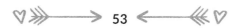

Ax-throwing

DATE: _____ / _____ / _____

If visiting a wreck room sounded a little too much, why not start with a more sedate evening down at the —er, local ax-throwing range?! It might not sound like your kind of thing, but giving ax-throwing a go is a great way of letting off some steam and testing your target-hitting skills together! Ax-throwing ranges can be found (often a little off the beaten track, admittedly!) in a lot of big towns and cities these days, and many are often paired with local bars and eateries so that you can make a day of it. And after a few practice throws (and a couple of drinks to steady your nerves, perhaps) maybe you'll even find you have a knack for it!

HOW DID IT GO?

DATE RATING: ♡ ♡ ♡ ♡ ♡

Fortune Telling

DATE: _____ / _____ / _____

No matter whether you're a believer or a skeptic, there's little denying fortune telling is often a fascinating curiosity. So why not give it a go by booking a session together with a local card reader or palm reader—or even a medium? It's up to you how you play this out and what your fortune-telling method of choice might be. It's also up to you too, of course, whether you choose to believe what you're told or take it all with a pinch of salt! Maybe it's best to reserve judgment, however, until after you've had your fortunes told and the predictions either start (or rather don't start!) to happen…?

HOW DID IT GO?

_____

_____

_____

_____

_____

DATE RATING: ♡ ♡ ♡ ♡ ♡

Visit a Microbrewery or Winery

DATE: _____ / _____ / _____

Popping out for a few drinks together every now and then is nothing new, of course, but what about taking the time to find out how those drinks are actually made? Microbrewing has become something of a buzzword in recent years, and small independent companies and premises have turned away from larger brewing brands to instead invest in making their own beers, ales, and similar drinks. Tracking one of these down—or, if beer is not your think, perhaps visiting a winery instead?—can make for a fascinating taste experience, as you get to sample different drinks and appreciate the differences, and all the hard work, that goes into them.

HOW DID IT GO?

_____

_____

_____

_____

_____

DATE RATING: ♡ ♡ ♡ ♡ ♡

Attend a Magic Show

DATE: ____ / ____ / ____

For many of us, seeing a magic show is probably something we last did at a friend's birthday party in childhood! But the performance doesn't end there, and many small-scale venues will often host magicians and illusionists who can put on just as dazzling a show for you in adulthood as you enjoyed as a kid. Search the local listings for a magic show in your area and pick up a couple of tickets for you and your partner to enjoy an evening of brain-bending illusionism and trickery. Who knows, you might even get invited up on stage to take part...

HOW DID IT GO?

_____

_____

_____

_____

_____

DATE RATING: ♡ ♡ ♡ ♡ ♡

Visit an Aquarium

DATE: ____ / ____ / ____

Aquariums and sea life centers are big summertime attractions for tourists and holidaymakers, of course, but even out of season—and even when they're on your own doorstep—these fascinating places are well worth a visit. If you're lucky enough to have an aquarium nearby, why not get yourselves a couple of tickets and drop in to learn more about the creatures of the deep and to see some truly bizarre and exotic animals? If your nearest aquarium is somewhat further afield, of course, you might need to factor a visit like this into a day trip or a vacation, in which case you can likely check off a few other date ideas along the way!

HOW DID IT GO?

_____
_____
_____
_____
_____

DATE RATING: ♡ ♡ ♡ ♡ ♡

Attend a Drag Show

DATE: ___ / ___ / ___

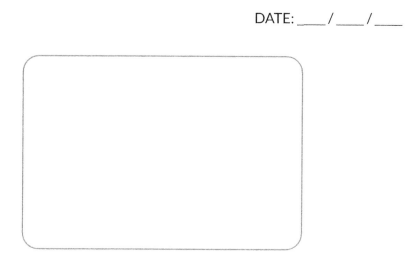

Since the arrival of *Ru Paul's Drag Race* on our screens in the early 2000s, drag shows have slipped into mainstream entertainment and can often now be found in clubs and venues of all shapes and sizes. Attending one is a great way of enjoying a form of entertainment you might never have seen or experienced anywhere before. In fact, you likely won't find this mixture of music, dancing, hilarious comedy roasting, and unadulterated glamor anywhere other than a drag show! Search your local comedy club listings for the next performance and get yourselves a pair of tickets for a fun night out on the town.

HOW DID IT GO?

_____
_____
_____
_____
_____

DATE RATING: ♡ ♡ ♡ ♡ ♡

Enjoy a Local Sunset Spot

Every town and city, no matter the size or location, will have some scenic hotspot from where to best watch the sun go down on a lazy summer's evening. It might be at the coast, out in the hills, away in the countryside, or even on a rooftop bar or restaurant—but putting in the time to find the best local sunset spot and get a date (weather dependent, of course!) fixed to go can be well worth the effort. If it's outdoors, remember to dress appropriately, and maybe take a drink or two with you to enjoy in the early evening twilight. Or, if it's at a local bar or similar venue, why not use this as an excuse to get all dressed up and really make a romantic night of it?

HOW DID IT GO?

_____

_____

_____

_____

_____

DATE RATING: ♡ ♡ ♡ ♡ ♡

Visit a Museum or Art Gallery

DATE: _____ / _____ / _____

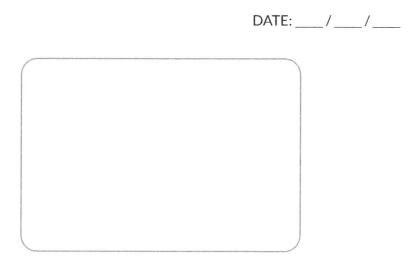

It's often tourists and school trips that make a beeline for local museums and art galleries—and if you're lucky enough to live somewhere where there are a plethora of cultural venues like these, it can be easy to take them for granted and never find the time to go. So why not find an exhibition of interest for you and your partner to visit? Some venues even host late-evening openings, where you can take the time to explore their collections after hours with a glass of wine and a canapé or two in hand!

HOW DID IT GO?

_____

_____

_____

_____

_____

DATE RATING: ♡ ♡ ♡ ♡ ♡

Go Birdwatching

Grab your binoculars and get out into the great outdoors to make the most of what our avian neighbors have to offer! Birdwatching or wildlife watching is a great way to not only get some much needed fresh air but to appreciate animals that we might never have given a second thought. Whether you're just heading to a local park or wildlife reserve or out into the mountains for a longer nature hike, be sure to read up on the kinds of birds and animals you might expect to see. Or why not make a game of it by writing out a checklist of, say, ten different species and seeing how many you can spot together?

HOW DID IT GO?

DATE RATING: ♡ ♡ ♡ ♡ ♡

Go Skating

Whether it's ice skating or roller blading, heading to the local skating rink is a sure-fire way to have some fun together. You don't even have to be a particularly accomplished skater to make the most of the day, either. Many rinks will organize classes for first-timers and unconfident beginners, but so long as you swallow your pride (and perhaps wear a good pair of gloves and some knee pads!) there's nothing to worry about if you're keen just to head out on your own. If you're already an experienced skater, of course, there's nothing to stop you and your other half from upping the romance by skating together for as long as you wish!

HOW DID IT GO?

DATE RATING: ♡ ♡ ♡ ♡ ♡

Go to a Gig or Concert

If you're a real music fan, chances are you're heading off to local gigs and concerts fairly regularly. But for the rest of us, work and modern life can often get in the way of enjoying live music—especially if we have to travel to a venue, or have work, kids, or pets to look after. Making the time to track down a band or artist both you and your partner like who is on tour in your area, however, can make for a great date night—especially if you have time beforehand to perhaps grab some food or a couple of drinks and really make the most of the evening! Don't forget to stop by the merch stand too on your way home...

HOW DID IT GO?

DATE RATING: ♡ ♡ ♡ ♡ ♡

Go to the Theater

DATE: _____ / _____ / _____

The theatre isn't for everyone, certainly—and for many of us, the last time we saw a live play or stage show was likely on a school English trip to see some Shakespeare! But if you're looking for a new cultural experience together, few things come close to the thrill of seeing a live theatrical performance, with the hushed energy of the crowd and the buzz of the actors stepping out onto the stage! Don't feel you need to limit yourself to a dramatic play, either. If Shakespeare isn't quite your thing, why not book tickets for a musical, a ballet or dance recital, or even an opera? Many larger theaters will have a schedule full of all kinds of shows, so take the time to find one that you are both keen to see and make an evening of it.

HOW DID IT GO?

_____
_____
_____
_____
_____

DATE RATING: ♡ ♡ ♡ ♡ ♡

Go to the Ballgame

DATE: _____ / _____ / _____

Some people are at the local stadium practically every other week—whereas for some of us, even the idea of seeing a live baseball or football game is something of our worst nightmare! But whether it's a regular occurrence or a one-off, seeing live sport together—amid the buzz of the crowd and the excitement of the game—is always a thrilling experience. Check out your local listings for live games in your area and get yourself a pair of tickets. Be sure to dress for the occasion, of course—not just in the colors of your team of choice, but in respect to the season too. You don't want to be wearing a T-shirt and shorts if you're, say, outside for three hours in the depths of winter!

HOW DID IT GO?

_____

_____

_____

_____

_____

DATE RATING: ♡ ♡ ♡ ♡ ♡

The Tourist Trap

Every town or city worth its salt will have its fair share of tourist attractions. But if that's your home town or home city, it's easy to walk past these local attractions without giving them a second thought. So why not take the time one day to visit one (or more!) of them together? Historical monument. Museum. Flea market. Concert hall. It's your choice what venue you choose. And why not book yourself onto a guided tour or join up with a tourist group to find out a little more about where you live and what it has to offer—and meet some new people along the way?

HOW DID IT GO?

DATE RATING: ♡ ♡ ♡ ♡ ♡

Bike Ride

DATE: ____ / ____ / ____

These days you don't even have to have a bicycle of your own to enjoy a nice relaxing bike ride in the countryside or along some local tourist route. Plenty of stores, workshops, and tourist centers will give you the chance to rent a bike for the day so that you can take in all the sights in the sunshine—while getting some fresh air and exercise too. Cycling is a great couple's activity too, giving you a chance to switch off from everything around you and spend time in peace and quiet with just you and your partner. Pick a route, pick a nice sunny day, and get pedaling!

HOW DID IT GO?

_____

_____

_____

_____

_____

DATE RATING: ♡ ♡ ♡ ♡ ♡

New Food Night

DATE: _____ / _____ / _____

It's all too easy for couples who have been together a long time to fall into a regular pattern of going to the same bars and restaurants every time they go out. Even couples who are just beginning their time together often find themselves choosing regular haunts and eateries they know well. But for something a little different, how about opting for a restaurant—and a cuisine—that neither of you have ever tried before? And then, once you're there, making a menu choice that is squarely outside of your comfort zone? It's a nice way of mixing things up on date night if you've been together a long time, and a nice way of seeing somewhere new—and experiencing it together—for couples who have only just met.

HOW DID IT GO?

_____
_____
_____
_____
_____
_____

DATE RATING: ♡ ♡ ♡ ♡ ♡

Scavenger Hunt

DATE: _____ / _____ / _____

Another idea that works just as well in adulthood as it likely did at school, a scavenger hunt is a hilarious activity for your next day out together. There are lots of ways to organize this, and it's up to you how the day pans out. Either one of you can set the hunt up for the other person, leaving clues around town for your partner to figure out. Perhaps make the last clue a hint to a venue, where you have been waiting all along for them to turn up! Alternatively, why not have a friend or another couple set up the hunt for you—or make this a group activity and have a few couples take part on the same day, leading you all to the same final venue?

HOW DID IT GO?

_____

_____

_____

_____

_____

DATE RATING: ♡ ♡ ♡ ♡ ♡

Play Pitch and Putt

DATE: _____ / _____ / _____

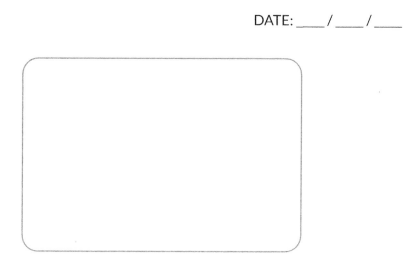

Whether it's crazy golf, mini golf, or pitch and putt, tackling a round together is a fun date idea for spending an afternoon or evening together in the sunshine. Pitch and putt requires relatively little skill (and is often more fun the less experienced a player you are!), and venues will let you rent clubs and balls. So all you need to do is find a golf range in your area, turn up, and start putting! First person to score a hole in one wins a bonus prize, of course...

HOW DID IT GO?

_____
_____
_____
_____
_____

DATE RATING: ♡ ♡ ♡ ♡ ♡

Go Thrifting and Antiquing

DATE: _____ / _____ / _____

Some towns and cities will have entire neighborhoods full of antique and thrift stores, which makes spending an afternoon exploring these old world stores for vintage finds and other treasures all the more simple. If you're not lucky enough to have a thrift store on your doorstep, however, keep an eye out for listings of vintage fairs and flea markets, which can offer just the same experience. No matter where you end up, wandering the aisles of antique stores and marketplaces is a fun and often fascinating day out and one that might end up with you bringing home one or two new (or rather old!) additions to your home!

HOW DID IT GO?

_____
_____
_____
_____
_____

DATE RATING: ♡ ♡ ♡ ♡ ♡

Silent Disco

Silent discos have come from nowhere in the last few years to become one of the hottest—if not, one of the strangest!—tickets in town. If you've never been to one before, the idea is simple: all the attendees wear headphones to listen and dance around to the music, so the disco itself remains silent while everyone there can hear the music played to them directly. It's a bizarre idea on paper but a great night out in reality—and well worth checking your local listings for one in your area for you and your partner's next date night!

HOW DID IT GO?

_____

_____

_____

_____

_____

DATE RATING: ♡ ♡ ♡ ♡ ♡

Murder Mystery Night

DATE: ____ / ____ / ____

These used to be all the rage in the 1980s and 90s before dying away (no pun intended!) when the internet and social media took over. Now seeing something of a retro resurgence, murder mystery evenings are a hilarious opportunity to pit your wits and nerve against a series of clues and situations, meet new people, and have a ball while doing it. You can either arrange your own mystery night and have you and your partner running the night while your friends solve the fictitious crime, download a plotline from the internet to solve together, or attend an organized murder mystery night (which are often hosted by local drama groups). Hunt around online for one in your area!

HOW DID IT GO?

_____
_____
_____
_____
_____

DATE RATING: ♡ ♡ ♡ ♡ ♡

Go Stargazing

DATE: ____ / ____ / ____

It used to be that you needed a top-of-the-range telescope and a degree or two in astrophysics to understand what is going on above you in the night sky, but these days you can rely on a geo-positioning app to decode the visible stars and planets above. You can also head out to a dark-sky park for an evening class or spot of stargazing with a professional. No matter how you choose to do it, going stargazing is a fascinating (and surprisingly romantic) activity! Just remember to dress warm if you're heading out in winter...

HOW DID IT GO?

_____

_____

_____

_____

_____

DATE RATING: ♡ ♡ ♡ ♡ ♡

Try Pet-sharing

Since the early 2000s, websites like CoPuppy and Borrow My Doggy have set non-pet owners up with vacationing or working pet owners, allowing those who have a dog but need to go out for the day—as well as those who do not have a dog but would love to!—to get in touch. If cats are more your thing (or, for that matter, rabbits, hamsters, gerbils, parrots, or anything else that takes your fancy!), pet sharing can be a fun experience as you get used to having an animal in your life, if only for a few hours or days at a time.

HOW DID IT GO?

_____

_____

_____

_____

_____

DATE RATING: ♡ ♡ ♡ ♡ ♡

Tree and Wildflower Hunting

DATE: _____ / _____ / _____

Going on a nature hike is one thing, but going out there with someone who knows the names of all the animals and plants you might walk by is another. Happily, these days you don't need your own park ranger to accompany you on a walk through the woods or a local country park—you can download an app or have a quick search online to find the kinds of flowers and trees you might encounter in your area at this time of year. List in hand, all you need to do is pick your location and go for a leisurely stroll together in the great outdoors and see how many you can check off as you go.

HOW DID IT GO?

_____
_____
_____
_____
_____

DATE RATING: ♡ ♡ ♡ ♡ ♡

Go to the Drive-in Cinema

DATE: ____ / ____ / ____

It's the most old-school date you can imagine: the drive-in cinema. They're not as popular (or, alas, as commonplace) as they used to be, but Hollywood has made the drive-in cinema a staple of all young lovers' courtships for decades now—so why don't you and your other half try continuing the tradition? If you don't have a drive-in in your local area, have a search for one-off outdoor cinema experiences and showings online to see if there's anything comparable. Then all you have to do is drive up, open the popcorn, and enjoy the film!

HOW DID IT GO?

_____

_____

_____

_____

_____

DATE RATING: ♡ ♡ ♡ ♡ ♡

Have a Spa Day

DATE: ____ / ____ / ____

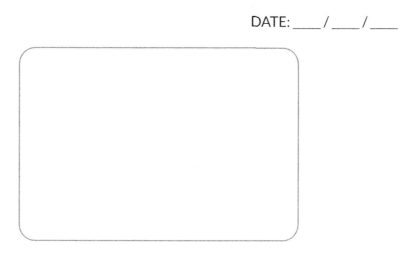

Admittedly, many couples today are so time-poor thanks to the rigors of work, commuting, kids, and other responsibilities that finding the time to do activities like those in this book is easier said than done. So why not try a date experience that will not only give you some quality time together but is designed especially to help you relax and unwind? A spa day is a great option for a couple who need a little rest and relaxation, as well as a few hours (or why not a weekend?!) away from everything else.

HOW DID IT GO?

_____

_____

_____

_____

_____

DATE RATING: ♡ ♡ ♡ ♡ ♡

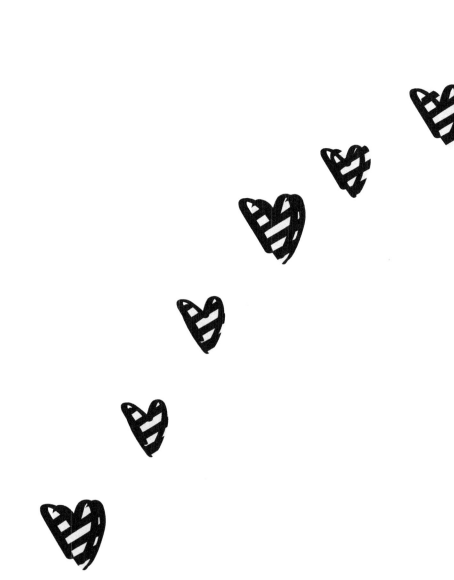

PART III

Take on the Challenge!

Try a Cookery Class

DATE: ____ / ____ / ____

Either with a one-off night class or a full week-by-week course, why not try improving your culinary skills together by attending a cookery class? Whether you're interested in just picking up the basics or are keen to learn something more ambitious, you should be able to find the class or the course for you in the local listings—many of which will be run in local cafes and bistros after closing hours.

HOW DID IT GO?

_____

_____

_____

_____

_____

DATE RATING: ♡ ♡ ♡ ♡ ♡

Try a Mixology Class

DATE: ____ / ____ / ____

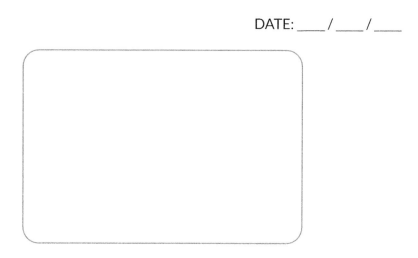

While we're on the subject of learning a new skill in the culinary and gastronomic world, why not try a mixology class too? Mixology is the "science" of making cocktails and other mixed drinks, and although most people will have a few recipes up their sleeve—the odd brunch-time Bloody Mary here, a summer barbecue's pitcher of margaritas there!—learning the techniques and ingredients involved in true classic cocktails can be a fun and enlightening experience. Take a look through local bar and restaurant listings online to find a class in your area and get yourselves booked in for a night!

HOW DID IT GO?

_____

_____

_____

_____

_____

DATE RATING: ♡ ♡ ♡ ♡ ♡

Learn a Language

DATE: _____ / _____ / _____

Let's be realistic here for a moment: you're not going to pick up a language to any level of fluency in a single class, or even in a few weeks' worth of lessons! But that's not the point here. Learning a language understandably takes time, but agreeing to tackle one together with your partner is a great way of not only learning a new skill but spending time together week after week. Night classes and conversation groups are a great way to start and are often listed in local newspapers and on school and church noticeboards. Whether it's something completely new to both of you or a high school skill you're trying to revive as an adult, pick the language you want to learn and get going!

HOW DID IT GO?

_____

_____

_____

_____

_____

DATE RATING: ♡ ♡ ♡ ♡ ♡

Take a Pottery Class

DATE: ____ / ____ / ____

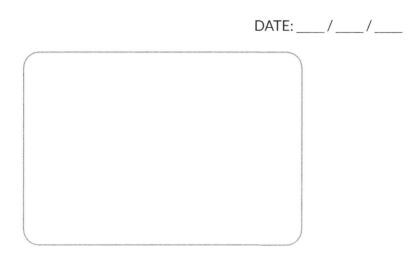

Another skill that has seen something of a resurgence in recent years is pottery. It used to be that only art students and those with wheels and kilns at home could take part in pottery, but these days pottery lessons can be found in community centers and school night classes—and even in high-street art shops and craft stores. So why not track down a class in your local area, and go and get your hands dirty!

HOW DID IT GO?

_____
_____
_____
_____
_____

DATE RATING: ♡ ♡ ♡ ♡ ♡

Attend a Wine Tasting

DATE: ____ / ____ / ____

Wine is one of those things that people who know a lot about it know A LOT about, while people who know little to nothing about it remain all but completely in the dark! Whether wine is a passion of yours or not, attending a wine tasting is a great way of finding out more about this fascinating and surprisingly complex subject and learning to appreciate the differences between different grapes, vineyards, and countries.

HOW DID IT GO?

_____

_____

_____

_____

_____

DATE RATING: ♡ ♡ ♡ ♡ ♡

Attend an Art Class

DATE: ____ / ____ / ____

Just like the pottery class of a page or two ago, attending an art class is a great way of exploring your creativity together—while having a great time in the process! No matter your own level of skill when it comes to drawing, painting, or sculpting (or whatever other art form you choose!), an art class is there to help you improve and explore this fascinating world. And who knows, you might turn out to be a natural!

HOW DID IT GO?

_____

_____

_____

_____

_____

DATE RATING: ♡ ♡ ♡ ♡ ♡

Attend a Comedy Night

DATE: ____ / ____ / ____

You can of course head down to your local comedy club any time you please—but instead of seeing a big-name comedian who's touring the length and breadth of the country, why not opt for something a little different? Open-mic nights and improv nights are always riotously good fun, with new and up-and-coming comedians testing out new material on smaller audiences and comic troupes taking madcap suggestions from the audience to create crazy scenarios live on the spot. Maybe just don't sit in the front row if you'd rather not end up part of the show…!

HOW DID IT GO?

DATE RATING: ♡ ♡ ♡ ♡ ♡

Take on a Trivia Night

DATE: ____ / ____ / ____

A staple midweek entertainment in pubs and bars all over the world, a trivia night or pub quiz can be a hilarious opportunity to not only tackle a question-and-answer challenge but find out how much your partner knows about anything and everything from First Ladies to the Seven Wonders of the World! Be sure to get there early to stake out a good table—and don't forget your pen!

HOW DID IT GO?

_____
_____
_____
_____
_____

DATE RATING: ♡ ♡ ♡ ♡ ♡

Head to the Driving Range

DATE: _____ / _____ / _____

Mark Twain once famously called a round of golf "a good walk spoiled." True, golf isn't for everyone—and if you're in Twain's group, the prospect of spending a few hours wandering around in the open slowly putting a ball ever closer to a hole probably doesn't sound too fun! The local driving range, however, offers something different. Whether you're a total novice or a seasoned pro, get yourself and your partner along for an evening of golf-swing practice. There's often equipment to borrow and coaches on hand to offer tips and advice should you need it.

HOW DID IT GO?

_____

_____

_____

_____

_____

DATE RATING: ♡ ♡ ♡ ♡ ♡

Try a Dance Class

DATE: ____ / ____ / ____

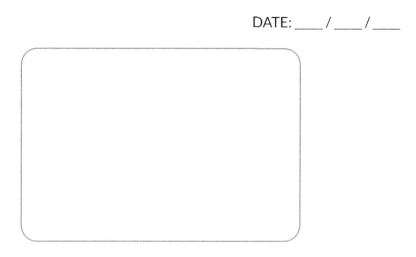

Ever since *Dancing with the Stars* became a hit, ballroom dancing classes have popped up all over the place—and this is your opportunity to try one out for yourself! Whether it's the tango or the smooth, the cha-cha or the Charleston, an instructor will guide you through the basic steps and have you and your partner dancing the night away within a matter of hours. If you enjoy it, you might even want to take up lessons together—but let's stick to the basics first...

HOW DID IT GO?

_____

_____

_____

_____

_____

DATE RATING: ♡ ♡ ♡ ♡ ♡

Go Geocaching

Another past fad that has seen a resurgence in popularity in recent years is geocaching. Using apps, maps, and global positioning equipment, players all over the world follow instructions to locate tiny containers—known as caches, or geocaches—that have been hidden everywhere from up trees and in caves to under park benches and inside post boxes. You can get involved simply by using an app or a similar online service, which will show you how many caches there are to find nearby. Think of it as like a kid's Easter egg hunt, except for adults!

HOW DID IT GO?

DATE RATING: ♡ ♡ ♡ ♡ ♡

Photographic Scavenger Hunt

DATE: _____ / _____ / _____

These days everyone has a camera on their smartphone, so this is a fun way of making the most of the tech at your fingertips. You can play either as a couple or as a group activity with other friends or couples: simply come up with a list of random objects or concepts, and give yourselves a time limit (an hour or two should be enough) before meeting back up in a bar or café to compare pictures. Make your target ideas as wild and as wacky as you like. Who will take the best picture of a giant letter H? A red balloon? An umbrella? A seahorse? A graffitied number? A broken window? Their own name that they've not written themselves? A selfie in an unexpected place? Make a list, get your camera at the ready, and start the timer!

HOW DID IT GO?

_____

_____

_____

_____

_____

DATE RATING: ♡ ♡ ♡ ♡ ♡

Try a Yoga Class

DATE: ____ / ____ / ____

Yoga, Pilates, and other stretching and callisthenic exercise classes have burst onto the fitness scene in the past few decades and remain as popular as ever today. If you've never tried one, the prospect of donning leggings and vests and getting into increasingly unwieldy positions on a mat in front of strangers might sound like a nightmare! But as any yoga fan will tell you, yoga groups and classes are always open to beginners and are a great way of improving your fitness while having fun and meeting new people. Plus your partner will be there for all the encouragement and moral support you might need!

HOW DID IT GO?

_____

_____

_____

_____

_____

DATE RATING: ♡ ♡ ♡ ♡ ♡

Find the Tallest Building

DATE: _____ / _____ / _____

If you live in a small town, this might be one that's worth keeping for your next trip to a big city ... but for those of you who already call a metropolis home, this bizarre challenge is often a lot more fun than it sounds! Take yourselves into the city center and try to find the tallest building you can. The aim is to take the highest photo you can—so try to find a building that not only permits tourists and visitors (so no tricking your way into an office or business premises!), but has a gallery or viewing platform offering a high-rise view of the city. Once you're there, snap your selfie together for a memento of your date!

HOW DID IT GO?

_____

_____

_____

_____

_____

DATE RATING: ♡ ♡ ♡ ♡ ♡

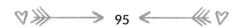

Try Meditation

This one works well alongside your yoga class. Track down a local meditation class and give you and your partner a well-earned break (and some much-needed thinking time) away from the hustle and bustle of modern life. Meditation classes are often organized by local religious centers and Buddhist groups, which are always welcome to new members keen to explore other cultures, regardless of their personal faith or belief. Think of this as just a chance to relax and unwind together in a way you might never have tried before.

HOW DID IT GO?

DATE RATING: ♡ ♡ ♡ ♡ ♡

Try Line Dancing

DATE: ____ / ____ / ____

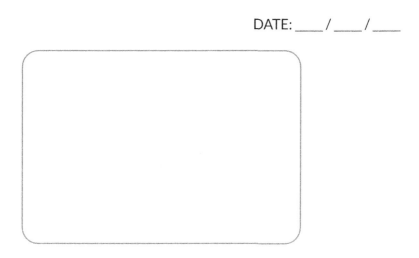

Get your cowboy boots at the ready and head to your local line dancing class for this date night challenge! Line dancing was a global trend in the late 90s and early 2000s, but if you're keen to take part you'll still find line dance evenings and classes easily enough if you just take a look on your local social listings. Often put on in bars and night clubs, a line dancing night is a hilarious test of you and your partner's coordination and musical skills—all while listening to some amazing country and western tunes!

HOW DID IT GO?

_____
_____
_____
_____
_____

DATE RATING: ♡ ♡ ♡ ♡ ♡

Get Out on the Water

DATE: ____ / ____ / ____

Interpret this one however you want—the goal is just to find an activity that is going to take you and your partner off dry land for an hour or so. That might be something adventurous, like trying wind surfing or paddle boarding, or it might be something more relaxing—like taking a pedal boat around the local park lake or buying a ticket for a pleasure cruise up and down the local riverside.

HOW DID IT GO?

_____
_____
_____
_____
_____

DATE RATING: ♡ ♡ ♡ ♡ ♡

Go Paintballing

DATE: _____ / _____ / _____

This works both as a date night activity or as a group with other like-minded and adventurous couples. Paintballing involves opposing teams aiming to score as many paint-filled shots against their opponents within the allotted time as they can. If you're playing as a pair, look for a venue that allows one-on-one paintballing, often around assault courses or in rooms and warehouses giving you plenty of places to hide! As a group, however, you can go paintballing out in the great outdoors, with games often played in forests and farmland. Either way, it's a great activity that not only pits you against your partner in a fun and original way but gives you a great adrenaline rush—and lots of exercise!

HOW DID IT GO?

_____
_____
_____
_____
_____

DATE RATING: ♡ ♡ ♡ ♡ ♡

Go Ghost Hunting

DATE: ____ / ____ / ____

Local historical societies often organize ghost walks and ghost-hunting evenings, especially around Halloween. Signing on to one of these is a great way of not only giving you and your partner a good spooky experience but learning more about the people and past of where you live. Besides taking a guided tour or, wandering the streets and haunted venues of wherever you happen to be, be sure to check listings for similar evenings in grand houses and manors, some of which put on ticketed ghost-hunting evenings for visitors and guests.

HOW DID IT GO?

_____

_____

_____

_____

_____

DATE RATING: ♡ ♡ ♡ ♡ ♡

Try Horse Riding

DATE: ____ / ____ / ____

The prospect of mounting and riding a horse might not be for everyone, of course, but whether this is something your're familiar with or a definite one-off, going horse riding is always a fun experience unlike any other. It's up to you (and your level of experience) to decide how this plays out. You might be a complete novice, in which case you and your partner might benefit from a visit to a local stables to have a nice, slow trot around a yard. Or for the more experienced, why not hire a horse for an hour or two and go for a leisurely canter around the local countryside and bridleways?

HOW DID IT GO?

_____
_____
_____
_____
_____

DATE RATING: ♡ ♡ ♡ ♡ ♡

Try Indoor Skydiving

DATE: ____ / ____ / ____

Another date night idea that quite simply did not exist a year or two ago, indoor skydiving is a thrill-seeker's chance to recreate the rush of jumping out of an airplane—without ever heading to the airport! Using powerful fans and turbines, indoor skydiving centers can blast you off the ground and keep you suspended in midair while you try turns, flips, and all the other tricks skydivers like to do—safe in the knowledge that the (heavily cushioned!) ground is just below you! Have a look online for your nearest venue.

HOW DID IT GO?

_____

_____

_____

_____

_____

DATE RATING: ♡ ♡ ♡ ♡ ♡

Take a Diving or Swimming Class

DATE: ____ / ____ / ____

No matter how confident you are in the water, taking on a swimming class—or, for the more experienced, a diving class—is a great way of improving your skills in the water and learning some new ones in the process. Sports centers, gymnasiums, and swimming pools often offer one-to-one and group classes, so take a look at their listings to see if anything sounds appealing and get yourselves booked!

HOW DID IT GO?

_____
_____
_____
_____
_____

DATE RATING: ♡ ♡ ♡ ♡ ♡

Visit a Botanical Garden

DATE: _____ / _____ / _____

A visit to a botanical garden is a little like taking a leisurely walk around some of the world's most beautiful and extraordinary natural creations. Think of it as like a zoo for plants and trees—so there are no nasty cages and enclosures! Botanical gardens are typically home to a vast array of plants and trees, from delicate and rare wildflowers to bizarre tropical trees, cacti, and palms. Wandering around can give us a fascinating and mind-boggling insight into the world around us—as well as make for a perfectly relaxing date experience!

HOW DID IT GO?

_____

_____

_____

_____

_____

DATE RATING: ♡ ♡ ♡ ♡ ♡

Confront Your Phobias

DATE: ____ / ____ / ____

So, what is it for you—spiders or heights? Crowds or birds? Enclosed spaces or open spaces? Everyone has that one bugbear that they detest and that fills them with dread at the mere thought of it! So what better way to tackle that phobia head on than with the support of your other half?! Depending on what your phobias are, you might be able to do this hand in hand—having your partner accompany you onto the viewing platform of a skyscraper if you're afraid of heights, for instance. Or if your phobias are more hardball, you could always attend a class or even a hypnotherapy session together to tackle the fear head on.

HOW DID IT GO?

_____

_____

_____

_____

_____

DATE RATING: ♡ ♡ ♡ ♡ ♡

Take on a New Sport

DATE: _____ / _____ / _____

No matter whether it's shuffleboard or boules, or croquet or archery, find a sport that neither you nor your partner have tried before and find a local venue that hosts it. Get yourselves booked onto a court or a class (or whatever the venue might be!) and tackle the challenge together. Most venues will supply all the equipment you need and will be happy to help with tips and playing advice if you ask. So just pick a sport and get playing!

HOW DID IT GO?

_____

_____

_____

_____

_____

DATE RATING: ♡ ♡ ♡ ♡ ♡

Try Trampolining

DATE: ____ / ____ / ____

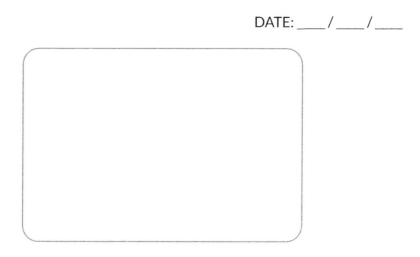

Trampolining is one of those things that if you don't try it as a kid, you've all but lost your chance to do so! Or at least, that's how it used to be. These days, trampolining parks and leisure centers offer everything from free-for-all sessions to one-to-one coaching, giving everyone the chance to try this most extraordinary (and extremely enjoyable) gymnastic sport. Don't worry if you've never tried it before, of course—whether you're a novice or a pro, the venue and the instructors will be on hand to make sure you take part in the safest way possible!

HOW DID IT GO?

_____

_____

_____

_____

_____

DATE RATING: ♡ ♡ ♡ ♡ ♡

Try Rock Climbing

DATE: ____ / ____ / ____

Much like trampolining, rock climbing is one of those activities that might seem out of reach (no pun intended) to many people. But in fact, climbing walls, abseiling lessons, and all manner of similar pursuits are often available at any local sports or outdoors center. No matter your level of fitness or experience—or, for that matter, how comfortable you are with heights!— there will be friendly staff and instructors on hand to make sure you have a good time and remain perfectly safe throughout.

HOW DID IT GO?

_____

_____

_____

_____

_____

DATE RATING: ♡ ♡ ♡ ♡ ♡

Conclusion

So how did it go?

We've come to the end of our Date Night Challenges here, and with 101 ideas now all attempted or completed, you've sure had a busy time of it getting to this last page!

Hopefully these last hundred pages or so have given you and your partner some experiences you'll never forget—and perhaps might never have thought to have had before! Even if all you got out of one of these experiences was a funny story or anecdote—or a mutual vow to, say, never be locked in an escape room ever again!—the point is that you tackled them together. And no matter whether you've checked all the boxes here or not (hey, rock climbing isn't for everyone!), you will still have made a hundred or so new memories along the way.

And maybe you've even picked up a few new skills or date ideas that you're going to take forward into the future and continue to use and participate in. Are you going to keep attending your art class or language class, for instance? Did the pottery throwing or wine tasting give you a new hobby? Or did swapping songs bring a new artist into your life that you now can't wait to see live together?

However your Date Night Challenges played out, all that remains is one final question. What challenge are you going to tackle together next?!

Printed in Great Britain
by Amazon

58047640R00066